# PRACTICAL INSULIN

## A HANDBOOK FOR PRESCRIBING PROVIDERS

### 6th Edition

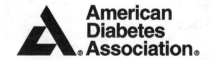

American
Diabetes
Association®

*Director, Book Operations,* Victor Van Beuren; *Assoc. Director/Managing Editor, Books,* John Clark; *Director, Book Marketing,* Annette Reape; *Writer,* Dr. Joshua Neumiller; *Composition,* Absolute Services; *Cover Design,* ADA; *Printer,* Lightning Source.

Printed in the United States of America

1 3 5 7 9 10 8 6 4 2

Nuha El Sayed, MD, MMSc, conducted the internal review of this book to ensure that it meets American Diabetes Association guidelines.

⊗ The paper in this publication meets the requirements of the ANSI Standard Z39.48-1992 (permanence of paper).

American Diabetes Association titles may be purchased for business or promotional use or for special sales. To purchase more than 50 copies of this book at a discount, or for custom editions of this book with your logo, contact the American Diabetes Association at the bulk book sales address below, at booksales@diabetes.org, or by calling 703-299-2046.

American Diabetes Association
Bulk Book Sales
PO Box 7023
Merrifield, Virginia 22116-7023

American Diabetes Association
2451 Crystal Drive, Suite 900
Arlington, VA 22202

DOI: 10.2337/9781580407632

Library of Congress Control Number: 2023938294

# Contents

# Introduction

JOSHUA J. NEUMILLER, PHARMD, CDCES, FADCES, FASCP
VICE-CHAIR & ALLEN I. WHITE DISTINGUISHED PROFESSOR
DEPARTMENT OF PHARMACOTHERAPY
COLLEGE OF PHARMACY AND PHARMACEUTICAL SCIENCES
WASHINGTON STATE UNIVERSITY
SPOKANE, WA, USA.

There is a good chance your practice is managing an ever-increasing number of people with diabetes. Insulin therapy is a medical necessity for all people with type 1 diabetes (T1D) and a useful treatment option for individuals with type 2 diabetes (T2D) who are unable to reach individualized glycemic targets with non-insulin glucose-lowering therapies. Understanding insulin products currently available on the market and current recommendations for use is vital to your practice and the people with diabetes under your care. Insulin's ability to lower glucose is unparalleled. Insulin both increases glucose uptake by tissues (muscle and adipose) and suppresses hepatic glucose release. The primary safety concern and limitation to insulin use is treatment-emergent hypoglycemia. In addition, insulin therapy can contribute to weight gain, a negative effect for people with T1D as well as for those with T2D who are often already struggling with overweight or obesity. In this handbook, you will find information on the many common questions and challenges involved in managing people with insulin—from choosing the best insulin regimen to meet individualized needs and preferences, to addressing reluctance to starting insulin therapy, to minimizing and/or preventing insulin-associated weight gain and hypoglycemia. As is true in the general management of diabetes, insulin therapy must be individualized to the needs and priorities of the person with diabetes, with no single insulin regimen or delivery device appropriate for all people with diabetes. Following recommended approaches to initiating and titrating insulin therapy in consideration of individualized treatment goals and based on glucose monitoring data will help you guide the person with diabetes to meet their management goals while also minimizing associated risks. The American Diabetes Association has published this sixth edition of *Practical Insulin: A Handbook for Prescribing Providers* in the hope that it will assist you as a clinical reference in your efforts to initiate and titrate insulin therapy to optimize outcomes for the people with T1D and T2D that you care for.

# Insulin: Basic Physiology and Pharmacology

Insulin is produced in the pancreas within the islets of Langerhans by β-cells and is secreted in response to rising blood glucose levels and neurohormonal signaling. When functioning normally, β-cells help maintain euglycemia via endogenous release of insulin to cover basal and prandial needs. In normal physiology, "basal insulin secretion" describes the low rate of insulin release between meals that is sufficient to inhibit overproduction of glucose and ketone bodies by the liver in the fasting state. Additional bursts of insulin are released to prevent hyperglycemia in the prandial state and promote conversion of nutrients to energy for short- and long-term use and storage (see **Figure 1**). Although **Figure 1** provides generalized statements related to physiologic insulin secretion during a given day, individual responses will vary.

Insulin action involves a complex series of responses that affect carbohydrate, lipid, and protein metabolism. Insulin carries out its metabolic and growth-promoting effects by binding to insulin receptors on cell plasma membranes. A key metabolic effect of insulin receptor activation is stimulation of glucose transport and metabolism. In the context of T1D, people have an absolute insulin deficiency and are unable to effectively transport and metabolize glucose. In people with T2D, the tissues are resistant to the effects of insulin, which leads to a relative insulin deficiency. Over time, pancreatic β-cells begin to fail in people with T2D as they continually work to produce more insulin to

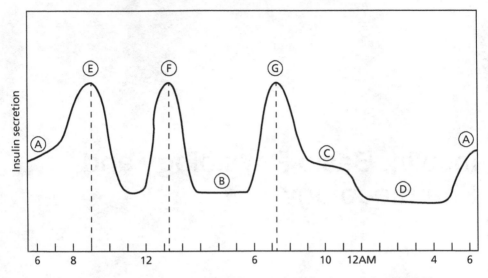

A: The dawn phenomenon starts at 4:00 A.M. and reaches its peak by 7:00–8:00 A.M. This peak is sustained until around 10:00 A.M., when levels fall. The dawn phenomenon may be a result of growth hormone and cortisol release, which begin to rise at 4:00 A.M., peak at 8:00 A.M., and fall at 10:00 A.M.

B: During the day in the fasting state, a small amount of basal insulin is released to maintain fasting glucose levels.

C: Because people are generally less active during the evening, insulin requirements tend to be slightly higher from 6:00 P.M. to 12:00 A.M. However, the increased insulin requirement is an individualized response.

D: The hormones are at their nadir from 12:00 A.M. to 4:00 A.M., so insulin requirements are lower.

E–G: Bursts of insulin are released from the pancreas to cover carbohydrate consumed with meals.

**Figure 1**—24-h normal physiologic insulin secretion.

counterbalance the persistent insulin resistance within the tissues. Eventually, β-cell function can decline to a level that requires exogenous insulin administration to achieve and maintain individualized glycemic targets. Although all insulin products work through activation of insulin receptors, their pharmacokinetic and pharmacodynamic profiles can vary significantly. The insulin primarily in use today is manufactured by way of recombinant DNA technology as either human insulin (**Figure 2**) or as rapid- or long-acting insulin analogs. Analog insulins are modified such that the amino acid sequence is intentionally altered to achieve the desired insulin action profile.

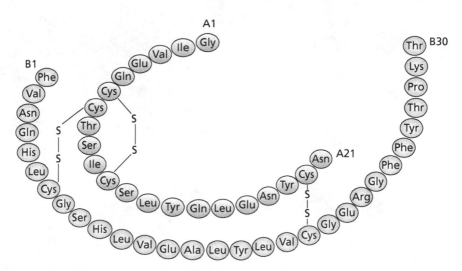

**Figure 2**—Structure of human insulin.

**Source:** Adapted from FeF Chemicals (available from: www.fefchemicals.com/biopharm/scientific-information/articles/the-insulin-peptide-family).

# Available Insulin Products

Insulin potency is measured in units, and the concentration of a given insulin product is expressed as units per milliliter. Various preparations sold in the United States (U.S.) at the time of this publication are available in U-100 (100 units/mL), U-200 (200 units/mL), U-300 (300 units/mL), and U-500 (500 units/mL) concentrations. U-500 regular insulin is generally reserved for people with T2D who have significant insulin resistance and take large daily doses of insulin, as discussed in the section *U-500 Regular Insulin*. **Table 1** summarizes key pharmacokinetic and pharmacodynamic properties of insulin products currently available in the U.S. The following sections discuss individual insulin products, as grouped by their general action profiles. A visual representation of the time-action profiles of currently available insulin products is provided in **Figure 3**.

## Rapid-Acting Insulin

Rapid-acting insulin is intended to mimic meal-stimulated insulin secretion as best as possible. The rapid onset of these insulin products improves our ability to match the insulin dose to carbohydrate intake and best align when insulin and glucose reach the circulation. Currently available injectable rapid-acting analogs (RAAs) include insulin aspart, insulin glulisine, and insulin lispro. RAAs are the insulin of choice for use in insulin pumps (see the section **INSULIN ADMINISTRATION AND USE CONSIDERATIONS** for

## Table 1—Summary of insulin pharmacokinetic and pharmacodynamic properties.*

| Product | | Time to onset of action (h) | Time to peak action (h) | Duration of action (h) |
|---|---|---|---|---|
| Generic name | Brand name(s) | | | |
| *Prandial (Mealtime) Insulin Products* | | | | |
| Aspart† | Novolog; Fiasp | within 0.25 | 0.5–1.5 | 4–6 |
| Glulisine | Apidra | within 0.25 | 0.5–1.5 | 4–6 |
| Lispro† (U-100, U-200) | Humalog; Admelog; Lyumjev | within 0.25 | 0.5–1.5 | 4–6 |
| Inhaled Human Insulin Powder† | Afrezza | within 0.25 | 0.5–1 | 1.5–4.5 |
| Regular Human Insulin (U-100) | Humulin R; Novolin R | 0.5 | 1.5–2.5 | 8 |
| *Intermediate-Acting Insulin* | | | | |
| NPH Insulin | Humulin N; Novolin N | 2–4 | 4–10 | 12–18 |
| *Long-Acting Insulin* | | | | |
| Detemir | Levemir | 2–4 | flat | 14–24 |
| Glargine (U-100) | Lantus; Basaglar; Semglee | 2–4 | flat | 20–24 |
| Glargine (U-300) | Toujeo | 6 | flat | up to 36 |
| Degludec (U-100, U-200) | Tresiba | 1 | flat | >42 |
| *Concentrated Regular Insulin* | | | | |
| Regular Human Insulin (U-500) | Humulin R U-500 | 0.5 | 4–8 | 13–24 |

* Person-specific onset, peak, and duration may vary from times listed in table. Peak and duration are dose-dependent with shorter durations of action seen for smaller doses and longer durations of action with larger doses.
† Insulin aspart and insulin lispro are available as multiple branded products—Fiasp, Lyumjev, and Afrezza have a relatively fast onset of action when compared to other rapid-acting insulin products.

additional information on insulin pump use). Injectable RAAs are engineered to dissociate and be absorbed more rapidly than regular human insulin (RHI), resulting in a faster onset and shorter duration of action. The faster onset of action allows for RAAs to be administered closer to the time of meal ingestion (typically 15 min before a meal), and the shorter duration of action lends to a reduction in between meal hypoglycemia. As an example, in one study,

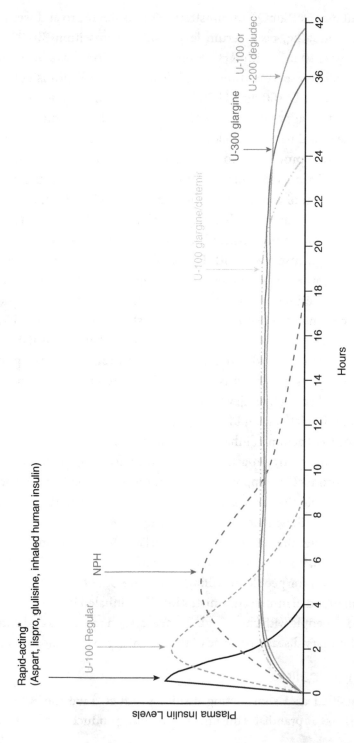

**Figure 3**—Insulin products by comparative action.

* Fiasp, Lyumjev, and Afrezza have a relatively fast onset of action when compared to other rapid-acting insulin products.

following subcutaneous (SubQ) administration of insulin lispro at doses ranging from 0.1–0.4 unit/kg, peak serum levels were seen within 30–90 min, compared with 50–120 min with RHI. Similar observations have been noted in studies with insulin aspart and insulin glulisine. Insulin lispro is commercially available in both U-100 and U-200 strengths, with a follow-on U-100 insulin lispro product approved by the U.S. Food and Drug Administration (FDA) under the brand name Admelog. Insulin aspart is likewise available as two different branded products: NovoLog and Fiasp. The faster-acting insulin aspart product (Fiasp) is formulated with niacinamide, which is believed to promote the formation of insulin monomers after SubQ injection, leading to more rapid absorption. Clinical trials comparing Fiasp and NovoLog in people with T1D and T2D showed a statistically significant improvement in lowering of 1-h postprandial glucose levels with Fiasp. Similarly, a faster-acting version of insulin lispro is now available under the brand name Lyumjev. These faster-acting agents are sometimes referred to as "ultra-rapid-acting insulin analogs." It is generally recommended that RAAs be administered no more than 15 min before a meal; however, it is acceptable for people to inject after a meal if carbohydrate intake is difficult to predict or if their rate of carbohydrate absorption is variable because of gastroparesis. It is possible that faster-acting insulin aspart (Fiasp) and insulin lispro (Lyumjev) products may have an advantage in this scenario due to their relatively rapid absorption profiles.

The mechanism of action of inhalable human insulin powder (brand name Afrezza), also classified as a rapid-acting insulin, differs from injectable rapid-acting insulins. The product is composed of insulin formulated in "microspheres" with a carrier molecule that allows insulin to be delivered into the deep lung for rapid absorption following inhalation (see **Figure 4**). Because of the rapid absorption in the lung, the onset of action is relatively faster than injectable RAAs. Inhaled human insulin is approved for use in people with T1D and T2D and is a viable option for people unwilling to initiate SubQ self-injection and can benefit from prandial insulin administration. This inhaled insulin product is contraindicated in people with chronic lung disease, such as asthma and chronic obstructive pulmonary disease, because of the risk of acute bronchospasm.

## Short-Acting Insulin

RHI is classified as a short-acting insulin product. Like the RAAs just discussed, RHI is a prandial (mealtime) insulin product used to cover

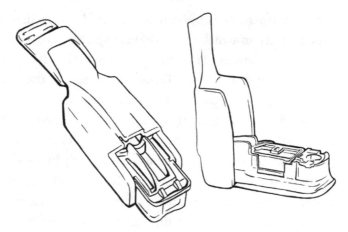

**Figure 4**—Afrezza inhalation device.

carbohydrate intake with meals. Compared with rapid-acting insulins, RHI has a slower onset and a longer duration of action (see **Table 1**). Following a single SubQ injection of 0.1 unit/kg of RHI to healthy subjects, peak insulin concentrations generally occur between 1.5 and 2.5 h post-dose, with insulin concentrations returning to baseline after ~5 h. The glucose-lowering effect of RHI starts ~30 min after SubQ administration; thus, RHI is typically injected 30–45 min before a meal to best match the expected postprandial rise in blood glucose. RHI administration through continuous intravenous infusion is often used for managing hyperglycemia in the critical-care setting. Although rapid-acting insulins have possible advantages related to their faster onset and shorter durations of action, RHI costs considerably less and can be used effectively in people unable to access newer analog insulin products. Of note, RHI can be purchased without a prescription at the pharmacy. A specific Walmart brand of RHI can be purchased without a prescription for approximately $25 per vial.

## Intermediate-Acting Insulin

Neutral protamine Hagedorn (NPH) insulin, also known as isophane insulin, is generally classified as "intermediate acting" in terms of its pharmacokinetic profile. NPH insulin contains an absorption-inhibiting substance called protamine, which prolongs the action and contributes to the cloudy appearance of NPH insulin. For this reason, NPH and NPH-type insulins (such as those contained in premixed insulin products) should be agitated or mixed before injection to resuspend the insulin mixture. NPH insulin may be used to cover basal insulin needs, in which case NPH is typically administered twice (sometimes three times) daily. NPH reaches peak plasma levels anywhere from 4–10 h after SubQ administration (see **Table 1**). Because of the notable peak with NPH insulin, its use is associated with higher rates of peak-dose hypoglycemia when compared with long-acting insulin analogs. Although NPH does carry a higher hypoglycemia risk, it is currently considerably less expensive than long-acting insulin analogs and can be used effectively in people who have difficulty obtaining more expensive insulin products. As discussed above for RHI, NPH insulin can be purchased without a prescription. Walmart also sells NPH insulin without a prescription for approximately $25 per vial.

## Long-Acting Insulin

Long-acting insulin products are basal insulin analogs that provide basal insulin coverage for up to 24 h or longer, depending on the product. Agents with a duration of action in excess of 24 h (U-300 insulin glargine and insulin detemir) are sometimes referred to as "ultra-long-acting" insulin products.

### Insulin Glargine (U-100)

Insulin glargine (U-100) differs structurally from human insulin by the addition of two arginines after position B30 and the replacement of asparagine with glycine at position A21. Unlike NPH insulin, insulin glargine is soluble at a pH of 4.0. Following SubQ injection, the acidic insulin solution is neutralized, leading to the formation of insulin microprecipitates from which small amounts of insulin are gradually released over time. As noted in **Table 1**, U-100 insulin glargine exhibits a duration of action generally ranging from 20–24 h with a relatively flat pharmacokinetic profile. In clinical trials, U-100 insulin glargine demonstrated similar effects on glycemic control when compared to once- or twice-daily NPH, with the advantage of a decreased rate of hypoglycemic events, particularly nocturnal hypoglycemia. In addition to the insulin glargine product Lantus, several follow-on U-100 insulin glargine products are available in the U.S., marketed as Basaglar and Semglee. Although some people can realize a full 24 h of basal coverage with a single injection of U-100 insulin glargine, some people require twice-daily administration for a full day of basal coverage.

## Insulin Detemir

Insulin detemir is another long-acting basal insulin analog. Insulin detemir has a prolonged duration of action (14–24 h) because of its ability to reversibly bind to albumin at the injection site and within the bloodstream. Structurally, insulin detemir differs from human insulin by the omission of threonine at position B30 and the attachment of myristic acid to lysine at position B29. The presence of myristic acid contributes to delayed dissociation and absorption of insulin detemir hexamers and facilitates a >98% binding of insulin detemir to albumin in the plasma and interstitial fluid. Because only free, non-albumin-bound insulin can be absorbed, albumin binding contributes to the prolonged duration of action seen with insulin detemir. Considering the duration of action of insulin detemir can range from 14–24 h, not everyone can realize a full 24 h of basal insulin coverage with once-daily administration. Twice-daily administration may be required in some people.

## Insulin Glargine (U-300)

U-300 insulin glargine is a three-fold concentrated version of insulin glargine. U-300 insulin glargine is similar to the U-100 product in terms of structure and solubility at an acidic pH of 4.0. The longer duration of action realized with the concentrated U-300 product is attributable to the smaller injection volume, which results in a smaller precipitate surface area. The smaller surface area results in a slower dissolution rate and a resultant longer duration of action (see **Figure 3**). Although the U-100 version of insulin glargine requires twice-daily administration in some people to achieve a full 24 h of basal coverage, once-daily administration of U-300 insulin glargine is sufficient to provide a full day of basal coverage. Because of the pharmacokinetic and pharmacodynamic properties of U-300 insulin glargine, time is needed for this insulin product to accumulate and reach steady-state levels, which generally are achieved after 5 days of once-daily administration. The manufacturer recommends titrating the dose no more frequently than every 3–4 days to minimize the risk of hypoglycemia.

Potential advantages of U-300 insulin glargine over the U-100 insulin glargine product include a longer duration of action, the potential for delivery of large insulin doses in a smaller injection volume, and a lower incidence of nocturnal hypoglycemia. Of note, when converting someone from the U-100 insulin glargine product to the U-300 product, larger doses (on a unit-per-unit basis) are typically needed to achieve the same glucose-lowering effect. Therefore, it can be expected that higher unit doses of U-300 insulin glargine will be required to maintain glycemic control compared with the previous U-100 insulin glargine dose.

## Insulin Degludec (U-100; U-200)

Insulin degludec is another long-acting basal insulin analog with a duration of action in the neighborhood of 42 h. Like U-300 insulin glargine, a single daily dose of insulin degludec will always provide sufficient coverage for a full 24 h. Steady-state insulin concentrations are achieved by 3–4 days of once-daily SubQ administration. To achieve this prolonged glycemic effect, insulin degludec is modified such that the amino acid at B30 is deleted and the lysine at position B29 is conjugated to hexadecanoic acid. When stored in solution with phenol and zinc, insulin degludec forms small, soluble, and stable dihexamers. Upon injection, the phenol component slowly dissipates, allowing for self-association of the insulin molecules into large multi-hexameric chains consisting of thousands of dihexamers connected to one another. Over time, these chains slowly begin to dissolve as the zinc component diffuses, resulting in the release of insulin from the terminal ends of the chain to be absorbed. Insulin degludec is commercially available in U-100 and U-200 concentrations. Unlike insulin glargine, variation in the concentration of insulin degludec does not alter its pharmacokinetic and pharmacodynamic properties. Thus, differences in the duration of action are not seen when comparing the U-100 and U-200 products. Like U-300 insulin glargine, the manufacturer recommends titrating the dose no more frequently than every 3–4 days to minimize the risk of hypoglycemia. Potential advantages of insulin degludec include its long duration of action, the potential for delivery of large insulin doses in a smaller injection volume (U-200 product), and a lower incidence of nocturnal hypoglycemia compared with U-100 insulin glargine. In addition, insulin degludec can be particularly useful in people with erratic schedules who may benefit from flexible dosing. Studies with insulin degludec have shown that dosing at variable times during the day has no impact on efficacy or hypoglycemia risk. It is recommended, however, that daily doses be separated by at least 8 h.

## U-500 Regular Insulin

U-500 regular insulin was first introduced in the U.S. in 1952 for use in people with extreme insulin resistance caused by antibody formation against animal-derived insulin products. Although a five-times concentrated RHI product, the pharmacokinetics of U-500 insulin are considerably different from U-100 RHI. U-500 insulin peaks around 30 min after SubQ injection and has a duration of action that can range widely (see **Table 1**). Historically, U-500 insulin use was associated with a high risk of insulin overdose errors with injection of U-500 with U-100 insulin syringes. In recent years, however, the availability of U-500 insulin pens and dedicated U-500 insulin syringes has improved the safety of this insulin product. Given the unique properties of U-500 insulin, its use is generally reserved for people with T2D with significant insulin resistance who take over 200 units of insulin daily. Following the publication of a U-500 clinical trial that used two dosing algorithms for the initiation and titration of U-500 in people with T2D who had not achieved adequate glycemic control with high-dose U-100 insulin therapy, dosing algorithms are now readily available to help guide clinicians in the use of U-500 insulin in people who could benefit from this product.

## Premixed Insulin Products

Some insulin products can be combined, or "mixed," in the same syringe to reduce the number of required daily injections. NPH or NPH-type insulin can be mixed with either RHI or rapid-acting insulin analogs. By mixing NPH-type insulins with regular insulin or a rapid-acting insulin analog, a biphasic action profile is created, providing both basal and prandial coverage with a single injection. When mixing insulins in a single syringe, the rapid- or short-acting insulin should be drawn up first. Note that long-acting insulins, such as insulin glargine, insulin detemir, and insulin degludec, should never be mixed with other insulin products in the same syringe. Due to the contemporary availability of premixed insulin products, people with diabetes in developed countries with good insulin access rarely need to mix insulins through use of vials and syringes.

Commercially available premixed insulin products contain set percentages of two types of insulins in the same solution. These include mixtures of NPH and RHI (70/30) and mixtures of protamine suspensions of RAAs with the respective RAA (75/25 lispro protamine/insulin lispro, 50/50 lispro prot-amine/insulin lispro, and 70/30 aspart protamine/insulin aspart). The primary advantages of these insulin products include convenience and accuracy of administration, particularly for people with vision or dexterity limitations for whom mixing insulin would be difficult or unreliable. In addition to fixed- dose insulin combination products, two currently available products combine a basal insulin analog with a glucagon-like peptide-1 (GLP-1) receptor agonist. Com-bination therapy with basal insulin and a GLP-1 receptor agonist can effectively target both fasting and postprandial glucose values and thus improve A1C and overall glycemic control while also mitigating insulin-associated weight gain. **Table 2** provides a summary of fixed-dose combination products available in the U.S. at the time of publication of this handbook.

# Table 2—Fixed-dose combination insulin products.

| Product | | Product Availability | Units per Pen | Dose Range per Injection (pens only) | Recommended Pen Storage at Room Temperature (days) |
|---|---|---|---|---|---|
| Generic Name | Brand Name(s) | | | | |
| *Fixed-Dose Combination Insulin Products* | | | | | |
| Regular/NPH 70/30 | Humulin 70/30 Novolin 70/30 | Vial, Prefilled pen | 300 units | 1–60 units | 10 |
| Lispro mix 50/50 | Humalog Mix 50/50 | Vial, Prefilled pen | 300 units | 1–60 units | 10 |
| Lispro mix 75/25 | Humalog Mix 75/25 | Vial, Prefilled pen | 300 units | 1–60 units | 10 |
| Aspart mix 70/30 | NovoLog Mix 70/30 | Vial, Prefilled pen | 300 units | 1–60 units | 14 |
| *Fixed-Dose Insulin/GLP-1 Receptor Agonist Products* | | | | | |
| Insulin Glargine/ Lixisenatide | Soliqua | Prefilled pen | 300 units (insulin glargine) | 15–60 units (insulin glargine) | 28 |
| Insulin Degludec/ Liraglutide | Xultophy | Prefilled pen | 300 units (insulin degludec) | 10–50 units (insulin degludec) | 21 |

# Insulin Administration and Use Considerations

W hen selecting an individualized insulin regimen for a person with diabetes, there are a variety of factors to consider. Such factors include, but are
not limited to cost and access considerations, self-management capabilities, and
person-specific treatment goals. On a product level, individual insulin products
are available in a variety of different delivery devices and have different recommendations for storage and use. **Table 3** provides a summary of current insulin
product availability and storage recommendations from the manufacturers. This
section will discuss several insulin use considerations, including the selection of
an insulin delivery method, key counseling regarding injection technique, and
insulin storage recommendations.

## Insulin Delivery Method

A variety of insulin delivery options are available. Options, in order of
increasing cost of use, include use of insulin vials and syringes (**Figure 5**), pens
with disposable cartridges, prefilled disposable pens (**Figure 6**), smart insulin
pens, and insulin pumps. The individual's resources as well as ability to prepare
and inject each insulin dose should be considered when recommending a delivery method.

## Table 3—Insulin Product Availability and Storage Information.

| Product | | | | | |
|---|---|---|---|---|---|
| Generic Name | Brand Name(s) | Product Availability | Units per Pen (if applicable) | Dose Range per Injection (pens only) | Recommended Pen Storage at Room Temperature (days) |
| *Prandial (Mealtime) Insulin Products* | | | | | |
| Insulin Aspart | NovoLog | Vial, Prefilled pen, Pen cartridges | 300 units | 1–60 units (FlexPen) 1–80 units (FlexTouch) | 28 |
| | Fiasp | Vial, Prefilled pen | 300 units | 1–80 units | 28 |
| Insulin Glulisine | Apidra | Vial, Prefilled pen | 300 units | 1–80 units | 28 |
| Insulin Lispro | Humalog (U-100) | Vial, Prefilled pen, Pen cartridges | 300 units | 1–60 units 0.5–30 units* | 28 |
| | Admelog (U-100) | Vial, Prefilled pen | 300 units | 1–80 units | 28 |
| | Humalog (U-200) | Prefilled pen | 600 units | 1–60 units | 28 |
| | Lyumjev (U-100) | Vial, Prefilled pen, Pen cartridges | 300 units | 1–60 units 0.5–30 units* | 28 |
| | Lyumjev (U-200) | Prefilled pen | 600 units | 1–60 units | 28 |
| Inhaled Human Insulin | Afrezza | Inhalation cartridges | N/A | N/A | N/A |
| Regular Human Insulin | Humulin R, Novolin R | Vial, prefilled pen | 300 units | 1–60 units | 28 |
| | Humulin R U-500 | Vial, Prefilled pen | 1,500 units | 5–300 units | 28 |
| *Intermediate-Acting Insulin Products* | | | | | |
| Human Insulin Isophane (NPH) | Humulin N Novolin N | Vial, Prefilled pen | 300 units | 1–60 units | 14 |

## Basal Insulin Products

| | | | | |
|---|---|---|---|---|
| Insulin Detemir | Levemir | Vial, Prefilled pen | 300 units | 1–60 units | 42 |
| Insulin Glargine (U-100) | Lantus | Vial, Prefilled pen | 300 units | 1–80 units | 28 |
| | Basaglar | Prefilled pen | 300 units | 1–80 units | 28 |
| | Semglee | Vial, Prefilled pen | 300 units | 1–80 units | 28 |
| Insulin Glargine (U-300) | Toujeo | Prefilled pen | 450 units (SoloStar) 900 units (Max SoloStar) | 1–80 units (SoloStar) 2–160 units (Max SoloStar) | 56 |
| Insulin Degludec (U-100, U-200) | Tresiba | Vial (U-100 only), Prefilled pen | 300 units (U-100) 600 units (U-200) | 1–80 units (U-100) 2–160 (U-200) | 56 |

**Abbreviations:** N/A, not applicable.
*KwikPen Junior.

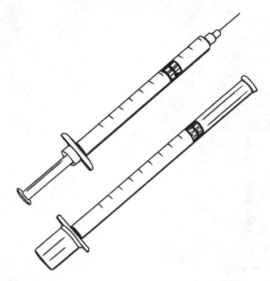

**Figure 5—**Insulin syringe.

## Vial and Syringe

Vials of insulin are generally less expensive than prefilled insulin pens or insulin cartridges. Many people can do quite well with vials and syringes, but use may be difficult for people with vision or dexterity limitations. People should be instructed to use a new, clean needle for every dose to prevent injection site infections. Insulin syringes are available in the U.S. for U-100 and U-500 insulin products. To prevent dosing and administration errors, U-200 and U-300 insulin products are available in pens only (see **Table 3**).

## Insulin Pens

Insulin pens provide a mode of delivery that is more convenient, and often more accurate, than insulin administration using a vial and syringe. These pens can be beneficial for people who have vision or dexterity issues that make the accuracy of drawing insulin into a syringe difficult. To prevent infection, a new disposable pen needle should be tightened on to the insulin pen before each use. Some of the pens also require priming the pen needle before each use and holding the needle in the injection site for a specific number of seconds, so manufacturer instructions should be explained to the person with diabetes before initiation.

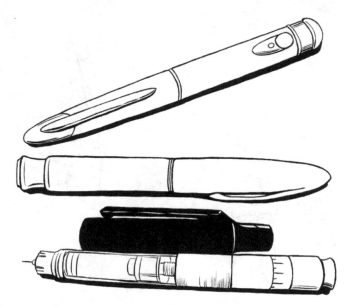

**Figure 6**—Insulin pens.

## Smart Connected Insulin Pens

Connected insulin pens have the capability of recording and/or transmitting insulin dosing information. Insulin pen caps are also available that can be placed on existing insulin pens to assist with calculating insulin doses. Some connected insulin pens and pen caps are programmable to help calculate insulin doses and provide downloadable data reports that can be shared with the diabetes care team to inform insulin dose adjustments. Use of connected insulin pens and pen caps require education to people with diabetes and/or their caregivers to ensure proper use.

## Continuous Subcutaneous Insulin Infusion (CSII; Insulin Pump)

Motivated people with T1D who desire increased flexibility with insulin administration may be candidates for continuous subcutaneous insulin infusion (CSII) through the use of an insulin pump. Most currently available insulin pumps deliver rapid-acting insulin through a SubQ cannula fed through tubing from the insulin pump (see **Figure 7**), while a few devices attach directly to the skin. Newer insulin pumps have the additional capability of interfacing with a continuous glucose monitor (CGM) to automate insulin delivery. Currently,

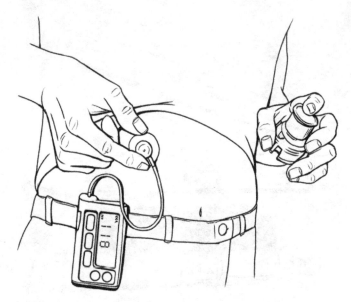

**Figure 7**—Insulin pump.

CSII is most frequently used in people with T1D because of limitations of insulin volume that can be loaded into an insulin pump. That said, insulin pumps are increasingly being used in the setting of T2D with the arrival of the V-Go patch pump that can deliver 24 h of insulin to people with T2D. CSII requires considerable education and support until the individual becomes familiar with use of the device. People initiating pump therapy should be referred for diabetes education sessions with a healthcare team that is experienced in pump therapy.

As previously noted, insulin pumps typically utilize rapid-acting insulin (insulin lispro, insulin aspart, or insulin glulisine) to cover both basal and bolus insulin needs (**Figure 8**). Insulin pump and patch technology advances quickly, with new-generation devices entering the market regularly. The American Diabetes Association's (The Association's) Diabetes Technology Guide website (https://diabetes.org/healthy-living/medication-treatments/diabetes-technology-guide) is an excellent resource for information on available diabetes technologies, including product functions and characteristics that may inform selection of a product that will best meet an individual's needs and priorities.

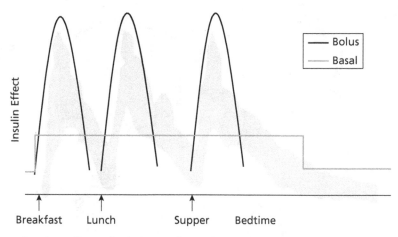

**Figure 8**—Insulin administration via an insulin pump.

## Injection Technique

Ensuring that people with diabetes and caregivers understand correct insulin injection technique is important to optimize glycemic outcomes and insulin use safety. Thus, it is important that insulin be delivered into the proper tissue in the right way. Proper insulin injection technique includes injecting into appropriate body areas, injection site rotation, appropriate care of injection sites to avoid infection or other complications, and avoidance of intramuscular (I.M.) insulin delivery.

Insulin should be injected into the SubQ tissue, not into an I.M. site. Recommended sites for insulin injection include the abdomen, thigh, buttock, and upper arm (**Figure 9**). Because insulin absorption from I.M. sites differs according to the activity of the muscle, inadvertent I.M. injection can lead to unpredictable insulin absorption and variable effects on glucose, with I.M. injection being associated with frequent and unexplained hypoglycemia. Risk for I.M. insulin delivery is increased in younger and lean individuals, when injecting into the limbs rather than truncal sites (abdomen and buttocks), and when using longer needles. Recent evidence supports the use of short needles (e.g., 4 mm pen needles) as being effective and well tolerated compared with longer needles, including a study performed in obese adults. Injection site rotation is also necessary to avoid lipohypertrophy and lipoatrophy. Lipohypertrophy appears as soft, smooth raised areas several centimeters in breadth and can contribute to erratic insulin absorption, increased glycemic variability,

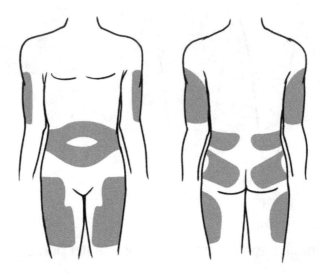

**Figure 9**—Insulin injection sites.

and unexplained hypoglycemic episodes. People using insulin should receive education about proper injection site rotation and learn to recognize and avoid areas of lipohypertrophy. Examination of insulin injection sites for the presence of lipohypertrophy, as well as assessment of injection device use and injection technique, are key components of a comprehensive diabetes medical evaluation and treatment plan. Numerous evidence-based insulin delivery recommendations have been published. Adherence to recommendations may lead to more effective use of this therapy and, as such, may hold the potential for improved clinical outcomes.

## Factors That May Affect Absorption

Several factors can affect the pharmacokinetic properties of insulin, regardless of insulin type. The site of injection, thickness of the SubQ tissue, amount of total body adipose tissue, SubQ blood flow, and amount of insulin administered all can affect the pharmacokinetics of exogenous insulin. Factors such as level of endogenous insulin secretion (T1D versus T2D) and obesity can also contribute to pharmacokinetic differences observed among individuals. Temperature variation can also have an influence on insulin absorption. Elevated skin temperature can lead to increased SubQ vasodilation, increasing blood flow to the injection site and causing insulin to be absorbed more rapidly.

Additionally, SubQ injections can be administered at multiple anatomic sites, such as the abdominal wall area, thigh, or upper arm. Most insulin manufacturers recommend rotating injection sites, but changing the anatomic site of injection can affect insulin absorption. People using insulin should be educated about factors that may influence insulin absorption when initiating insulin therapy and periodically thereafter. The following factors may be considered to facilitate more predictable absorption:

- **Injection site:** Potential SubQ injection sites include the abdomen (avoiding 1–2 inches around the navel), upper thighs, hips and buttocks, or back of the upper arms. However, injections into the abdomen, with its larger overall blood circulation and higher body heat, provide the quickest and most predictable absorption of rapid-acting and regular insulin. Avoidance of edematous sites is advised.

- **Injection site rotation:** People with diabetes can choose one body area for injection and rotate within that area or can rotate among body areas. Systematic rotation helps prevent lipohypertrophy, a result of insulin stimulation of fat cell growth, which delays insulin absorption. If people develop sites of lipohypertrophy, they should avoid injecting into these areas.

- **Injection volume:** Variability in insulin absorption is increased and net absorption is decreased as the volume of insulin in a single injection increases. For individuals with significant insulin resistance who are using large doses of insulin, smaller injections given multiple times per day may help decrease the variability in absorption. Using concentrated insulin products is another approach that can be used to decrease injection volume.

- **Blood flow:** Practices that increase regional blood flow (e.g., exercise, local massage or friction, hot showers, or soaks and saunas) can speed the absorption of insulin and thus alter insulin action.

## Insulin Storage

Unopened vials, cartridges, and pens of insulin should be refrigerated when not in use and should be used before the labeled expiration date. Once opened, insulin vials can be stored at room temperature. While in use, insulin pens should never be stored with a pen needle attached to prevent contamination of the insulin. Encourage people with diabetes to follow the manufacturer's recommendations for storing open insulin pens and/or cartridges (see **Table 2** and **Table 3**).

Exposure to freezing, direct sunlight, or high temperatures will decrease insulin potency. Instruct people to examine insulin appearance before injection. NPH insulin should appear uniformly cloudy without clumping or sediment after gentle resuspension; rapid-, short-, and long-acting insulins should appear clear without any particulates in the insulin solution. Counsel people not to use insulin if the appearance is not correct and to contact their pharmacist or provider for further advice and guidance.

# General Approaches and Recommendations for Insulin Use in People with Diabetes

Among all available glucose-lowering strategies, intensive (basal/bolus) insulin therapy has the greatest absolute potential for lowering A1C. The degree to which glycemia can be reduced with intensive insulin therapy is limited only by hypoglycemia. Unlike many other glucose-lowering medications that target either fasting plasma glucose or postprandial glucose, insulin can be used to target fasting glucose, postprandial glucose, or both, depending on the needs of the individual. Given the risks of hypoglycemia and weight gain, however, the risks and benefits of insulin treatment must be considered against those of other treatment approaches in people with T2D.

The following sections provide a general discussion of approaches to insulin use in people with T1D and T2D. While this information may be helpful in understanding generally recommended approaches to insulin use in these populations, the information provided is by no means the only approach to successfully initiating and titrating insulin in people with diabetes.

## Type 1 Diabetes

Exogenous insulin therapy is a requirement for people with T1D because of a lack of endogenous insulin secretion from pancreatic β-cells. As such, all people with T1D should be managed with an intensive insulin regimen designed to cover both basal and prandial (mealtime) insulin needs, with the ultimate goal of achieving individualized glycemic goals. Indeed, the Diabetes Control and Complications Trial (DCCT) showed that an intensive treatment strategy with multiple daily injections (MDI) or CSII resulted in improved glycemic control and better long-term outcomes in people with T1D. Therefore, people with T1D are ideally managed on an intensive MDI insulin regimen or use of CSII.

| Injected insulin regimens | Flexibility | Lower risk of hypoglycemia | Higher costs |
|---|---|---|---|
| MDI with LAA + RAA or URAA | +++ | +++ | +++ |

Less-preferred, alternative injected insulin regimens

| | | | |
|---|---|---|---|
| MDI with NPH + RAA or URAA | ++ | ++ | ++ |
| MDI with NPH + short-acting (regular) insulin | ++ | + | + |
| Two daily injections with NPH + short-acting (regular) insulin or premixed | + | + | + |

| Continuous insulin infusion regimens | Flexibility | Lower risk of hypoglycemia | Higher costs |
|---|---|---|---|
| Hybrid closed-loop technology | +++++ | +++++ | ++++++ |
| Insulin pump with threshold/ predictive low-glucose suspend | ++++ | ++++ | +++++ |
| Insulin pump therapy without automation | +++ | +++ | ++++ |

**Figure 10**—Representative relative attributes of insulin delivery approaches in people with T1D.[1]

*Legend:* Continuous glucose monitoring improves outcomes with injected or infused insulin and is superior to blood glucose monitoring. Inhaled insulin may be used in place of injectable prandial insulin.

[1]The number of plus signs (+) is an estimate of relative association of the regimen with increased flexibility, lower risk of hypoglycemia, and higher costs between the considered regimens.

*Abbreviations:* LAA, long-acting insulin analog; MDI, multiple daily injections; RAA, rapid-acting insulin analog; URAA, ultra-rapid-acting insulin analog.

An intensive basal/bolus regimen in someone with T1D is generally inclusive of a long-acting insulin that mimics normal basal insulin release seen in people without diabetes where ~1 unit of insulin is secreted every hour to handle the fasting insulin needs of the liver and muscle. A rapid-acting insulin is also administered in conjunction with the ingestion of carbohydrates at mealtimes, which simulates the rapid release of insulin from the pancreas that typically occurs in the fed state. Similarly, CSII allows for the infusion of rapid-acting insulin to cover both basal and prandial insulin needs (**Figure 8**). The approach to insulin delivery selected should consider the priorities, preferences, and capabilities of the person with T1D (**Figure 10**).

The Association makes the following specific recommendations pertaining to insulin therapy in people with T1D:

- Most people with T1D should be treated with multiple daily injections of prandial insulin and basal insulin or CSII.
- Most individuals with T1D should use rapid-acting insulin analogs to reduce hypoglycemia risk.
- Individuals with T1D should receive education on how to match mealtime insulin doses to carbohydrate intake, fat and protein content, and anticipated physical activity.

## Glycemic Goals and Targets in People with Type 1 Diabetes

As noted previously, treatment goals and expectations should be individualized for all people with diabetes, including those with T1D. **Table 4** summarizes general glycemic recommendations for nonpregnant adults with diabetes. Goals for children and adolescents should likewise be individualized per recommendations and considerations provided by the Association

## Table 4—Glycemic recommendations for many nonpregnant adults with diabetes.

| A1C | <7.0%* |
|---|---|
| **Fasting (Preprandial) Glucose** | 80–130 mg/dL* |
| **Postprandial Glucose** | <180 mg/dL* |

*More or less stringent glycemic goals may be appropriate in individuals.

within the *Standards of Care in Diabetes*. While general recommendations for A1C and blood glucose levels are provided, a variety of person-specific factors should be considered when establishing individualized goals and targets. Factors that may inform glycemic goals include risk of hypoglycemia and other adverse drug events, diabetes disease duration, life expectancy, comorbidity burden, presence of vascular complications, attitudes and treatment expectations of the individual, and resources and support available to implement a given treatment plan. When glycemic goal setting in children and adolescents with T1D, the Association outlines the following key considerations:

- Goals should be individualized, and lower goals may be reasonable based on a benefit-risk assessment.
- Blood glucose goals should be modified in children with frequent hypoglycemia or hypoglycemia unawareness.
- Postprandial blood glucose values should be measured when there is a discrepancy between preprandial blood glucose values and A1C levels and to assess preprandial insulin doses in those on basal/bolus or CSII regimens.

Ultimately, the Association recommends that treatment decisions and glycemic goal setting should be made in collaboration with the individual, whenever possible, to incorporate their needs, preferences, and values.

## Insulin Initiation and Titration

When initiating insulin therapy in someone newly diagnosed with T1D, the starting insulin dose is generally calculated based on weight, with starting doses typically ranging from 0.4–1.0 unit/kg/day of total insulin. The *American Diabetes Association/JDRF Type 1 Diabetes Sourcebook* notes 0.5 unit/kg/day as a typical starting dose when the person is metabolically stable, with subsequent titration of the insulin per glycemic response. After calculating the total daily insulin dose, approximately half of the calculated total daily dose is administered as basal insulin, with the other half distributed across meals as prandial insulin (such as one-sixth of the total daily dose injected at breakfast, lunch, and dinner, for example). Note that this weight-based total daily dose calculation and allocation is a starting point only and should be subsequently adjusted according to individualized insulin needs. The following provides an example total daily insulin dose–calculation in a person recently diagnosed with T1D:

**Example 1:** RJ is a 60-kg person recently diagnosed with T1D. It is decided that a total daily dose of 0.5 unit/kg/day is an appropriate starting point.

- **Total Daily Dose** = 60 kg × 0.5 unit/kg/day = *30 units/day*
- **Basal Dose** = 30 units/2 = *15 units of basal insulin daily*
- **Prandial Insulin** = Remaining 15 units/3 meals = *5 units of prandial insulin per meal*

Of note, there is no one gold standard method for initiating insulin in people with T1D. Although the previous example provides a starting point for insulin initiation, the weight-based dose calculation is an estimation of insulin needs only. For example, in people with T1D who are still in the honeymoon phase, lower weight-based doses of insulin may initially be needed until all endogenous insulin production has ceased. The basal and prandial insulin doses will inevitably require adjustment to meet individualized glycemic goals. Blood glucose monitoring and/or CGM are important tools to evaluate an insulin regimen and inform insulin titration decisions. Ideally, people with T1D will learn to count carbohydrates and adjust insulin doses based on carbohydrate intake and also will utilize insulin correction doses to correct for residual hyperglycemia before meals and potentially at bedtime. In the short term, however, fixed-dose prandial insulin can be used effectively until the individual is able to correctly count carbohydrates and adjust insulin doses based on meal content. Fixed dosing may also be a safer strategy in those with limited self-care capabilities, such as those unable to reliably count carbohydrates. The following section provides specific information on establishing an insulin-to-carbohydrate (I:C) ratio.

## *Insulin-to-Carbohydrate (I:C) Ratios*

Ideally, prandial (mealtime) insulin doses are precisely calculated in people with T1D to cover the amount of carbohydrate to be consumed. A typical ballpark I:C ratio in someone with T1D is 1:10 (1 unit of prandial insulin to cover 10 g of carbohydrate) or 1:15. These are estimates, however, and each person's needs vary. For people taking RAAs to cover meals, the "500 Rule" provides a reasonable initial estimate for determining a person's I:C ratio. To use the 500

Rule, the current total daily dose of insulin is simply divided into 500 to determine an estimated I:C ratio.

**Example 2:** SR, a person with T1D, is currently taking 30 units of U-100
insulin glargine once daily and a total of 20 units of insulin aspart divided
among breakfast, lunch, and dinner. His total daily insulin dose is 50 units.
SR would like to begin adjusting his mealtime insulin doses using an I:C ratio.

- **The 500 Rule:** 500/total daily insulin dose = 500/50 = 10
- **Interpretation:** 1 unit of insulin aspart will cover ~10 g of carbohydrate consumed with meals.
- **Application:** SR is planning to consume 40 g of carbohydrate at
  lunch. Using his estimated I:C ratio, he will inject 4 units of insulin
  aspart before the meal. SR was advised to check his blood glucose
  before the meal and 2 h after the meal to assess and reevaluate the
  appropriateness of his I:C ratio estimate.

## Correction Doses

Correction doses are important when blood glucose levels are unexpectedly
elevated. A correction factor is ultimately used to correct for a glucose reading
in the hyperglycemic range before meals or at bedtime, as examples. The "1800
Rule" is another simple calculation that can be used in people using RAAs at
meals. The calculation estimates how far 1 unit of rapid-acting insulin will drop a
person's glucose. To use the 1800 Rule, the number 1,800 is divided by the total
daily dose of insulin to determine the individual's correction factor. The following example shows how to use the 1800 Rule to estimate a correction factor:

**Example 3:** MJ is currently taking 30 units of U-100 insulin glargine once
daily and an average total of 30 units of insulin aspart divided among breakfast, lunch, and dinner after recently implementing an I:C ratio of 1:10. His
total daily insulin dose is ~60 units. MJ would now like to determine his
correction factor to better control his glucose throughout the day.

- **The 1800 Rule:** 1,800/total daily insulin dose = 1,800/60 = 30.
- **Interpretation:** 1 unit of insulin aspart will drop MJ's glucose by
  an estimated 30 mg/dL.
- **Application:** MJ is about to consume 40 g of carbohydrate at
  lunch. His premeal blood glucose reading is 160 mg/dL (his goal

premeal blood glucose is 100 mg/dL). Using his I:C ratio, he will administer 4 units to cover carbohydrates, and using his correction factor, he will administer an additional 2 units of insulin to account for the 60 mg/dL he is above his target premeal glucose. In total, MJ will administer 6 units of insulin aspart before lunch.

### Ongoing Insulin Adjustment in T1D

Although a variety of tools and estimates can be used to initiate and titrate insulin in people with T1D, the job of optimizing insulin therapy is an ongoing and iterative process. Insulin needs can and will change based on numerous factors. Illness, stress, diet, physical activity, and even the changing of the seasons can have dramatic effects on glycemic control and insulin needs. Using information obtained from blood glucose monitoring and/or CGM can be extremely valuable in pinpointing glycemic trends and making adjustments to diet, physical activity, and/or insulin doses to improve glucose management. People with T1D should be encouraged and empowered to take an active role in identifying trends and factors that affect their glucose to improve self-management skills and outcomes. For additional information and recommendations related to the overall management of people with T1D, please refer to the Association's Position Statements *Type 1 Diabetes in Adults* and *Type 1 Diabetes in Children and Adolescents* as well as the section on *Children and Adolescents* within the Association's *Standards of Care in Diabetes*.

## Type 2 Diabetes

The approach to insulin use in people with T2D is quite different from the approach taken in people with T1D. Although people with T1D initiate an intensive insulin regimen shortly after diagnosis, people with T2D can often be managed successfully with non-insulin therapies for years before the addition of insulin is required to meet individualized glycemic goals. That said, many people with T2D can benefit from early basal insulin initiation, depending on individualized needs and preferences. Once people with T2D reach the point at which they are not achieving individualized glycemic goals despite the use of multiple non-insulin glucose-lowering therapies, they may need to progress to use of injectable therapies. **Figure 11** provides recommendations from the Association's *Standards of Care in Diabetes* regarding treatment intensification to injectable therapies in people with T2D. As highlighted in **Figure 11**, if

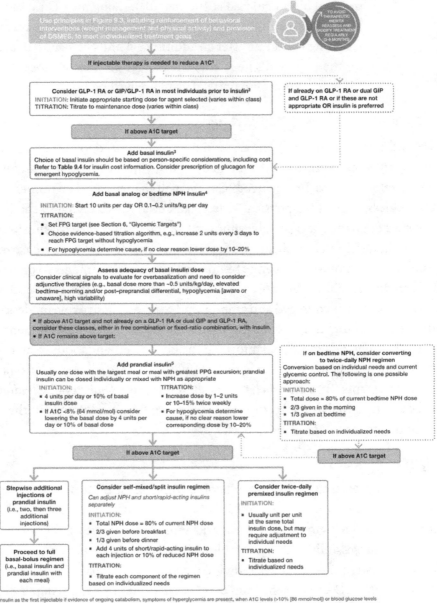

Use principles in Figure 9.3, including reinforcement of behavioral interventions (weight management and physical activity) and provision of DSMES, to meet individualized treatment goals

TO AVOID THERAPEUTIC INERTIA REASSESS AND MODIFY TREATMENT REGULARLY (3–6 MONTHS)

**If injectable therapy is needed to reduce A1C[1]**

**Consider GLP-1 RA or GIP/GLP-1 RA in most individuals prior to insulin[2]**
INITIATION: Initiate appropriate starting dose for agent selected (varies within class)
TITRATION: Titrate to maintenance dose (varies within class)

If already on GLP-1 RA or dual GIP and GLP-1 RA or if these are not appropriate OR insulin is preferred

**If above A1C target**

**Add basal insulin[3]**
Choice of basal insulin should be based on person-specific considerations, including cost. Refer to Table 9.4 for insulin cost information. Consider prescription of glucagon for emergent hypoglycemia.

**Add basal analog or bedtime NPH insulin[4]**
INITIATION: Start 10 units per day OR 0.1–0.2 units/kg per day
TITRATION:
- Set FPG target (see Section 6, "Glycemic Targets")
- Choose evidence-based titration algorithm, e.g., increase 2 units every 3 days to reach FPG target without hypoglycemia
- For hypoglycemia determine cause, if no clear reason lower dose by 10–20%

**Assess adequacy of basal insulin dose**
Consider clinical signals to evaluate for overbasalization and need to consider adjunctive therapies (e.g., basal dose more than ~0.5 units/kg/day, elevated bedtime–morning and/or post–preprandial differential, hypoglycemia [aware or unaware], high variability)

- If above A1C target and not already on a GLP-1 RA or dual GIP and GLP-1 RA, consider these classes, either in free combination or fixed-ratio combination, with insulin.
- If A1C remains above target:

**Add prandial insulin[5]**
Usually one dose with the largest meal or meal with greatest PPG excursion; prandial insulin can be dosed individually or mixed with NPH as appropriate

INITIATION:
- 4 units per day or 10% of basal insulin dose
- If A1C <8% (64 mmol/mol) consider lowering the basal dose by 4 units per day or 10% of basal dose

TITRATION:
- Increase dose by 1–2 units or 10–15% twice weekly
- For hypoglycemia determine cause, if no clear reason lower corresponding dose by 10–20%

**If on bedtime NPH, consider converting to twice-daily NPH regimen**
Conversion based on individual needs and current glycemic control. The following is one possible approach:
INITIATION:
- Total dose = 80% of current bedtime NPH dose
- 2/3 given in the morning
- 1/3 given at bedtime
TITRATION:
- Titrate based on individualized needs

**If above A1C target**          **If above A1C target**

**Stepwise additional injections of prandial insulin** (i.e., two, then three additional injections)

**Proceed to full basal-bolus regimen** (i.e., basal insulin and prandial insulin with each meal)

**Consider self-mixed/split insulin regimen**
Can adjust NPH and short/rapid-acting insulins separately

INITIATION:
- Total NPH dose = 80% of current NPH dose
- 2/3 given before breakfast
- 1/3 given before dinner
- Add 4 units of short/rapid-acting insulin to each injection or 10% of reduced NPH dose

TITRATION:
- Titrate each component of the regimen based on individualized needs

**Consider twice-daily premixed insulin regimen**
INITIATION:
- Usually unit per unit at the same total insulin dose, but may require adjustment to individual needs
TITRATION:
- Titrate based on individualized needs

1. Consider insulin as the first injectable if evidence of ongoing catabolism, symptoms of hyperglycemia are present, when A1C levels (>10% [86 mmol/mol]) or blood glucose levels (300 mg/dL [16.7 mmol/L]) are very high, or a diagnosis of type 1 diabetes is a possibility.
2. When selecting GLP-1 RA, consider individual preference, A1C lowering, weight-lowering effect, or fequency of injection. If CVD is present, consider GLP-1 RA with proven CVD benefit. Oral or injectable GLP-1 RA are appropriate.
3. For people on GLP-1 RA and basal insulin combination, consider use of a fixed-ratio combination product (IDegLira or iGlarLixi).
4. Consider switching from evening NPH to a basal analog if the individual develops hypoglycemia and/or frequently forgets to administer NPH in the evening and would be better managed with an A.M. dose of a long-acting basal insulin.
5. If adding prandial insulin to NPH, consider initiation of a self-mixed or premixed insulin regimen to decrease the number of injections required.

# Figure 11—Intensifying to injectable therapies in type 2 diabetes.

injectable therapy is needed to reduce A1C, it is recommended that a GLP-1 receptor agonist be considered as the first injectable agent in most people with T2D. Insulin is recommended as the first injectable in those with a very high A1C (>10%), those with symptoms or evidence of catabolism (e.g., weight loss, polyuria, polydipsia), or if a diagnosis of T1D is a possibility. The figure provides some guidance on the initiation and titration of basal insulin, inclusive of a recommended starting dose (10 units/day or 0.1–0.2 units/kg/day) and guidance on titration of the basal insulin to achieve an individualized fasting glucose target. If the goal A1C is not met following basal insulin optimization and achievement of the target fasting glucose level, the addition of a GLP-1 receptor agonist (if one is already not a component of the regimen) or prandial insulin is recommended. Prandial insulin is recommended to be started at 4 units/day or 10% of the basal dose typically initiated once daily with the largest meal (or meal with the largest postprandial glucose excursion). The dose can be up-titrated by 1–2 units or 10–15% twice weekly, with dose reductions of 10–20% recommended in the presence of hypoglycemia. Depending on response, additional injections of prandial insulin can be added until individualized glycemic goals are achieved. Although **Figure 11** provides a framework for insulin initiation and titration in people with T2D, individual needs will vary, and strategies should be individualized to meet glycemic goals and minimize hypoglycemia. **Figure 12** provides additional considerations for managing concomitant oral glucose-lowering medications once injectable therapies are initiated.

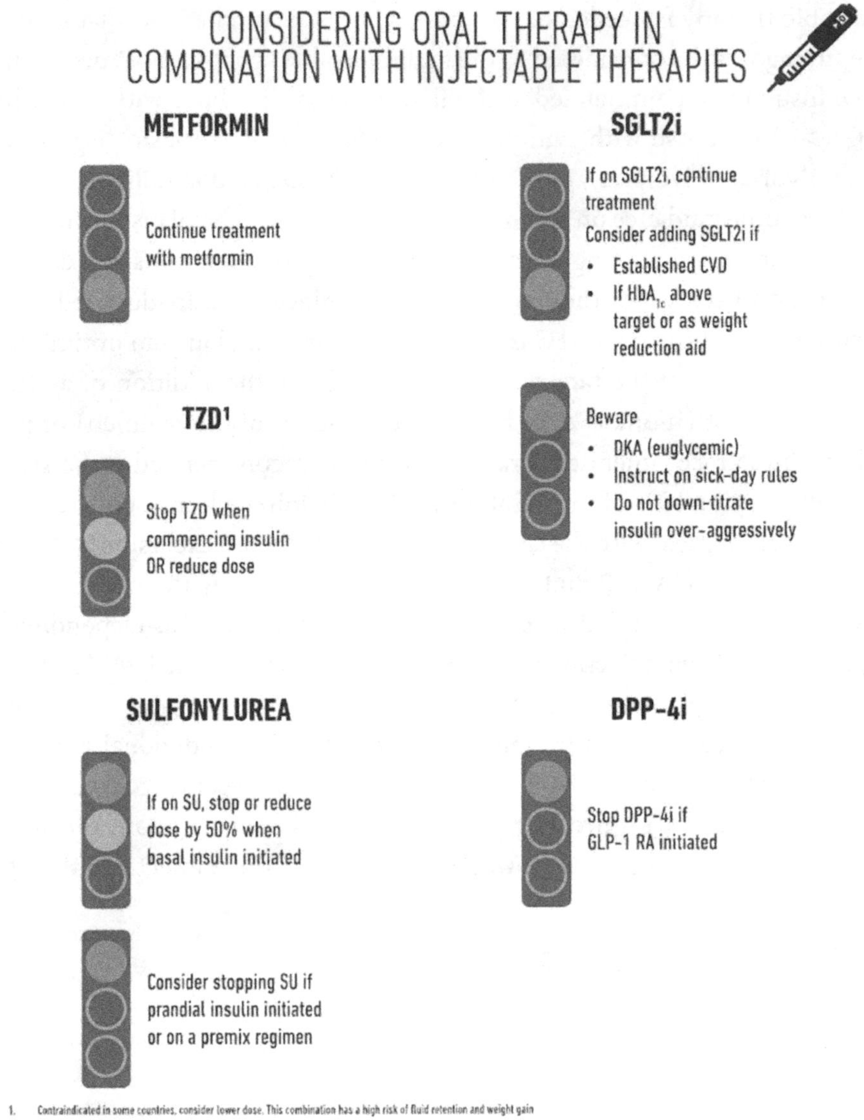

# CONSIDERING ORAL THERAPY IN COMBINATION WITH INJECTABLE THERAPIES

## METFORMIN

Continue treatment
with metformin

## TZD[1]

Stop TZD when
commencing insulin
OR reduce dose

## SULFONYLUREA

If on SU, stop or reduce
dose by 50% when
basal insulin initiated

Consider stopping SU if
prandial insulin initiated
or on a premix regimen

## SGLT2i

If on SGLT2i, continue
treatment
Consider adding SGLT2i if
• Established CVD
• If HbA$_{1c}$ above
  target or as weight
  reduction aid

Beware
• DKA (euglycemic)
• Instruct on sick-day rules
• Do not down-titrate
  insulin over-aggressively

## DPP-4i

Stop DPP-4i if
GLP-1 RA initiated

1.   Contraindicated in some countries, consider lower dose. This combination has a high risk of fluid retention and weight gain

**Figure 12**—Considering oral therapy in combination with injectable therapies.

# Sample Insulin Regimens

People with T1D will generally be on a regimen consisting of multiple daily injections or use of an insulin pump, but insulin regimens can vary dramatically in people with T2D. The following discussion reviews select insulin regimens and their respective advantages and disadvantages.

## Two Injections per Day

*Regimen:* Mixed or premixed insulin: RHI plus NPR or RAA plus isophane mix (e.g., lispro mix 50/50) (**Figure 13** and **Figure 14**).

*Theory:* Postprandial glucose levels for the morning and evening meals are covered by short- or rapid-acting insulin; lunch and overnight glucose levels are covered by NPH/isophane.

*Advantage:* Provides some basal and mealtime coverage with only two injections per day.

*Disadvantages: 1)* NPH given at the evening meal peaks during the night and often does not last overnight until breakfast, leading to potential nocturnal hypoglycemia or high pre-breakfast glucose levels. *2)* There is a lack of flexibility in dealing with midday glucose levels because the NPH dose and resultant action time are set at breakfast based on expectations of food and activity for the day. It would be unlikely that a person with T1D could achieve adequate glucose control with this regimen.

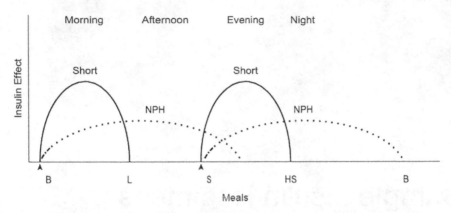

**Figure 13**—Two injections per day.

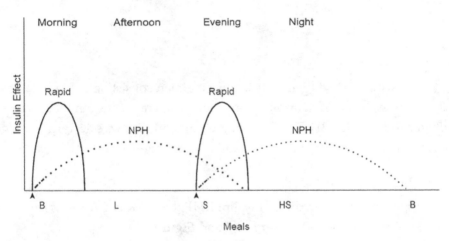

**Figure 14**—Two injections per day.

## Three Injections per Day

*Regimen:* Three injections per day using NPH and an RAA or short-acting insulin before breakfast, rapid-acting or short-acting insulin at the evening meal, and NPH at bedtime (**Figure 15** and **Figure 16**).

*Theory:* Same advantages as discussed for two injections per day, except that administering NPH at bedtime rather than at the evening meal may better control glucose levels overnight.

*Advantage:* Better overnight glucose control compared with a twice-daily premixed regimen.

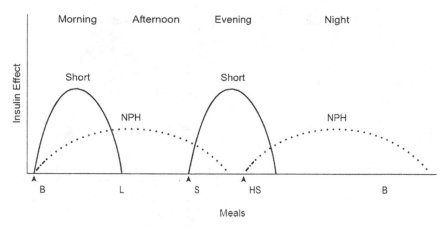

**Figure 15**—Three injections per day.

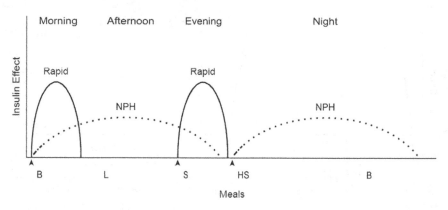

**Figure 16**—Three injections per day.

*Disadvantages: 1)* There is a lack of flexibility in dealing with midday glucose levels after lunch. *2)* This approach would require separate insulin products and could not be administered with a premix product alone. Again, it would be unlikely that a person with T1D could achieve adequate glucose control with this regimen.

## Four Injections per Day, Example 1

*Regimen:* Four injections per day using rapid-acting insulin analog plus twice-daily NPH or a long-acting insulin analog (**Figure 17** and **Figure 18**).

*Theory:* Two doses of NPH or one or two doses of long-acting insulin provide basal coverage during the day and overnight. Rapid-acting insulin covers postprandial glucose with each meal.

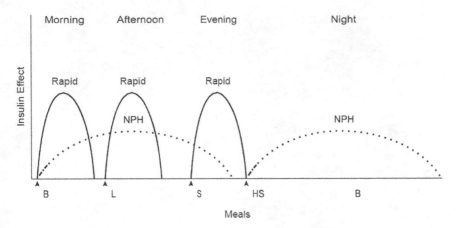

**Figure 17**—Four injections per day, example 1.

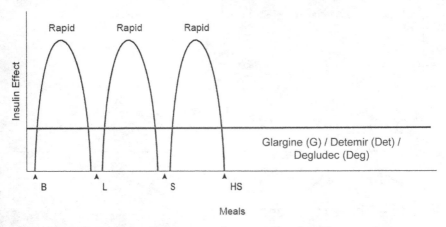

**Figure 18**—Four injections per day, example 1.

*Advantages:* Allows meal-to-meal adjustments of insulin dose based on pre-prandial glucose levels, carbohydrate intake, and activity and permits greater freedom of timing for meals.

*Disadvantages for NPH-containing regimen: 1)* NPH given in the evening peaks during the night and often does not last overnight until breakfast, leading to potential nocturnal hypoglycemia or high pre-breakfast glucose levels. *2)* Initial injection at breakfast requires mixing the NPH and rapid-acting insulins.

## Four Injections per Day, Example 2

*Regimen:* Four injections per day using short-acting insulin and twice-daily NPH or a long-acting insulin analog (**Figure 19** and **Figure 20**).

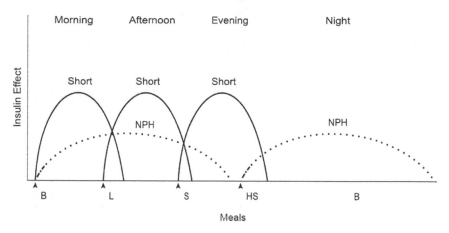

**Figure 19**—Four injections per day, example 2.

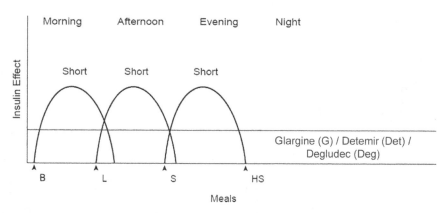

**Figure 20**—Four injections per day, example 2.

*Theory:* Short-acting insulin provides daytime and meal glucose control, and one dose of long-acting insulin analog or twice-daily NPH provides basal coverage during the day and overnight.

*Advantage:* Allows meal-to-meal adjustments of insulin based on prepran-dial glucose levels, carbohydrate intake, and activity.

*Disadvantage:* The long duration of regular insulin may lead to delayed between-meal and overnight hypoglycemia.

# Troubleshooting Barriers to Insulin Use and Key Adverse Events

Although intensive (basal/bolus) insulin therapy is unmatched in terms of glucose-lowering potential, its use comes with risks of hypoglycemia, weight gain, and injection site reactions. Initiation of insulin therapy inherently comes with a requirement for more intensive medical oversight and training related to proper insulin use and administration. These considerations can lead to hesitance to initiate insulin on the part of both people with diabetes and health-care providers alike.

## Barriers to Insulin Use in Type 2 Diabetes

Many people with T2D are good candidates for insulin therapy, but the person with diabetes and/or their provider may be resistant to initiating insulin therapy despite rising glucose levels for fear of complicating the therapy or concerns regarding hypoglycemia. Education is the key to increasing provider knowledge and comfort with using insulin. Providers who are comfortable with insulin therapy are more apt to gain acceptance from the person with diabetes when insulin therapy is indicated. Education and positive support are key components to effective and safe use of insulin.

Suggestions to increase knowledge and acceptance of insulin therapy for people with T2D include the following:

- Provide education and ensure understanding that the disease course includes progressive loss of β-cell function, and that insulin therapy is generally an expected treatment over time, not a sign of failure on the part of the person with diabetes.
- Avoid using the prospect of insulin therapy as a threat to increase adherence to lifestyle change or other therapies.
- Reinforce the short-term benefits of improved glycemia, including decreased nocturia and improved energy levels.
- Reinforce or reintroduce information about the importance of optimizing glucose management to preserve health and improve overall well-being and prevent long-term diabetes-related complications.
- Suggest that the person with diabetes try a bedtime injection routine of insulin glargine, detemir, degludec, or NPH for 1–2 months, and then plan to discuss whether they feel better and have more energy.
- Point out that newer needles make insulin therapy essentially painless and much more convenient than before, and discuss alternatives to syringes, such as insulin pens.
- Provide or refer the person with diabetes for diabetes self-management education that covers handling and filling syringes, strategies to maximize comfort with injections, as well as ongoing self-management support.

## Hypoglycemia

Hypoglycemia is the most common and serious adverse event associated with insulin use. Hypoglycemia is defined generally as a blood glucose value <70 mg/dL, with lower blood glucose levels associated with progressively severe hypoglycemic symptoms. Hypoglycemia is much more common with the use of prandial insulin products. Careful and methodic titration of basal insulin can minimize hypoglycemia risk, although overbasalization can contribute to hypoglycemic events. Signs of overbasalization include a basal insulin dose above 0.5 units/kg/day, elevated bedtime-to-morning and/or post-to-preprandial differential, and/or high glycemic variability. Because people with T1D are managed with intensive insulin regimens, they are generally at greater overall risk for hypoglycemia. That said, some people with T2D also receive intensive insulin therapy and should be considered high risk for hypoglycemic events, particularly when insulin is used in combination with sulfonylureas or other insulin secretagogue medications. Use of insulin in combination with insulin sensitizers (such as thiazolidinediones) may also increase risk.

All people who use insulin should be counseled regarding the signs, symptoms, prevention, and proper treatment of hypoglycemia. Although not exhaustive, **Table 5** provides a list of potential hypoglycemic symptoms. Mild hypoglycemia can be treated by following the "rule of 15": treat with 15 g carbohydrate, wait 15 min, and then check the blood glucose level. If after 15 min the blood glucose remains <70 mg/dL, another 15 g of carbohydrate should be consumed. Once the blood glucose is normalized, a snack or meal including complex carbohydrates and protein should be consumed to prevent a secondary hypoglycemic episode. When a severe hypoglycemic event occurs and glucose cannot be delivered orally, glucagon is indicated. The Association's *Standards of Care in Diabetes* recommends that glucagon be prescribed to individuals at significant risk of severe hypoglycemia, which would include people

## Table 5—Symptoms of hypoglycemia.

- Shakiness
- Nervousness or anxiety
- Sweating, chills, or clamminess
- Irritability or impatience
- Confusion, including delirium
- Rapid or fast heartbeat
- Lightheadedness or dizziness
- Hunger and nausea
- Sleepiness
- Blurred or impaired vision
- Tingling or numbness in the lips or tongue
- Headaches
- Weakness or fatigue
- Anger, stubbornness, or sadness
- Lack of coordination
- Nightmares
- Seizures
- Unconsciousness

who use prandial insulin products. Newer glucagon formulations—including intranasal and ready-to-inject glucagon—offer products with increased ease of use when compared to traditional glucagon injection powder kits. People with diabetes, their caregivers, and school personnel (if applicable) should all be educated on appropriate glucagon administration and use in the case of a hypoglycemic emergency.

## Hypoglycemia Unawareness

Some people with diabetes lose their ability to recognize normal warning symptoms of hypoglycemia, or the symptoms are blunted or absent. These individuals are at high risk for severe hypoglycemia. Hypoglycemia unawareness develops more commonly in people with T1D who have frequent hypoglycemic episodes and have had diabetes for many years. Preventing hypoglycemia can help reverse hypoglycemia unawareness. The Association states that people with hypoglycemia unawareness who experience one or more severe hypoglycemic events may benefit from at least short-term relaxation of glycemic targets so that their awareness and counter-regulation can be improved. Hypoglycemia awareness training can also improve recognition of early manifestations of hypoglycemia and prevent severe hypoglycemic episodes. People with hypoglycemia unawareness are particularly suitable candidates for use of CGM to detect and prevent hypoglycemic events. People at risk should additionally receive education about prevention and safety, including more frequent glucose monitoring, particularly before driving or other potentially hazardous activities. Because people with hypoglycemia unawareness are at high risk for severe hypoglycemia, they should receive a prescription for glucagon, with appropriate counseling and education on use provided to the individual and their family members or caregivers.

## Weight Gain

Insulin use is associated with weight gain. As glycemic control improves, glucose is utilized by the tissues instead of being lost in the urine, thus resulting in weight gain. Although insulin-associated weight gain is initially viewed as desirable in people with T1D because of the weight loss experienced secondary to glucosuria and catabolism that is frequently present at the time of diagnosis, intensive insulin therapy can result in undesirable weight gain over time. Indeed, some people with T1D may even underdose insulin as a strategy to avoid weight gain. For those with T2D, who often struggle with overweight and obesity, insulin therapy can further contribute to weight gain. Use of prandial insulin in people with T2D generally contributes to more weight gain than the use of basal insulin products alone. Both hypoglycemia treatment and possibly increased caloric intake in defense against hypoglycemia can contribute to weight gain. People starting insulin therapy should be informed of the potential for weight gain and be encouraged to implement healthy lifestyle measures to minimize insulin-induced weight gain. In people with T2D, adjunctive glucose-lowering agents, such as GLP-1 receptor agonists, SGLT2 inhibitors, and pramlintide, can be used for their insulin-sparing and weight-mitigating effects. Medications approved by the FDA for weight loss can also be considered.

## Adjustments for Physical Activity

When initiating an exercise routine, it can be useful to encourage people with diabetes to exercise at the same time every day, for a consistent duration, and at a similar intensity, to facilitate consistent therapy adjustments that will reduce the risk of severe hypoglycemia. This is particularly helpful for people with T1D. In addition, glucose monitoring before and after exercise will help identify necessary changes in food or insulin intake and educate the person with diabetes about his or her individual glycemic response to particular physical activities. For people using CGM, CGM data can be incredibly helpful to visualize the effects of physical activity on glucose levels. Once people understand how to adjust their insulin and food intake in relation to physical activity, they will be better able to anticipate the adjustments needed for varying types and durations of physical activity.

The following recommendations apply primarily to people with T1D; however, if a person with T2D experiences exercise-induced hypoglycemia, these same recommendations can be helpful:

- When the person plans to exercise after a meal, begin by cutting the meal-related rapid- or short-acting insulin dose. If the person with diabetes is unfamiliar with the glycemic effect of a given activity and the activity is more strenuous, reduce the dose by half. Use glucose monitoring results to determine whether the lowered dose resulted in hyperglycemia, glucose values within the desired target range (e.g., 80–130 mg/dL), or hypoglycemia. If needed, adjust up or down by 3% of total daily insulin requirements to prepare for a similar bout of exercise (i.e., similar in timing, duration, intensity).

- When the individual plans to exercise before eating, they may need to eat supplementary carbohydrates. This is a simpler option than reducing the prandial insulin dose before a meal.

# Education and Resources for People with Diabetes

Perhaps the most important aspect of diabetes care is the relationships between the person with diabetes and the members of their diabetes care team. One essential element of this partnership is empowering persons with diabetes through self-management education. Encourage people with diabetes to learn all they can about how to successfully manage their diabetes, including appropriate insulin dose adjustments in response to meals, physical activity, and blood glucose monitoring results. Stress the importance of actively engaging in their diabetes self-management, including glucose monitoring, record-keeping, healthy eating, and engaging in appropriate levels of physical activity. Healthy living with diabetes is largely driven by an individual's efforts at diabetes self-management.

A wide variety of educational materials are available from the American Diabetes Association targeting the needs of people living with diabetes. The American Diabetes Association Call Center can be reached at 1-800-DIA-BETES and people can visit the American Diabetes Association website at www.diabetes.org to access a wide range of educational resources and tools.

The American Diabetes Association has a wide variety of medical management publications for healthcare professionals, such as the following books:

*Medical Management of Type 1 Diabetes; Medical Management of Type 2 Diabetes; Intensive Diabetes Management; Medical Management of Pregnancy*

*Complicated by Diabetes;* and the *Guide to Medications for the Treatment of Diabetes Mellitus.*

For more information on these and other professional titles published by the American Diabetes Association:

- Visit the American Diabetes Association online bookstore at www.shopdiabetes.org
- Call 1-800-232-6733
- Visit any nationwide bookseller

## Appendix 1 – Sample blood glucose and medication log.

| Date | Time | Breakfast | Medicine/Comment | Time | Lunch | Medicine/Comment | Time | Dinner | Medicine/Comment | Time | Snack/Other | Medicine/Comment |
|------|------|-----------|------------------|------|-------|------------------|------|--------|------------------|------|-------------|------------------|
|      |      |           |                  |      |       |                  |      |        |                  |      |             |                  |
|      |      |           |                  |      |       |                  |      |        |                  |      |             |                  |
|      |      |           |                  |      |       |                  |      |        |                  |      |             |                  |
|      |      |           |                  |      |       |                  |      |        |                  |      |             |                  |
|      |      |           |                  |      |       |                  |      |        |                  |      |             |                  |
|      |      |           |                  |      |       |                  |      |        |                  |      |             |                  |

# Index

Note: Page numbers followed by an *f* refer to figures. Page numbers followed by *t* refer to tables.

## A

A1C (glycated hemoglobin $A_{1c}$)
   intensive insulin therapy and, 29
   in type 1 diabetes, 31*t*, 32
   in type 2 diabetes, 35–37
Absorption, 26–27
Admelog, 8*t*, 10, 20*t*. *See also* Insulin lispro
Administration, 19–28
   delivery methods for, 19–24, 20*t*–22*t*
   injection sites for, 25–26, 26*f*
   injection techniques for, 25–26
   pens for, 19, 22–23, 23*f*
   pumps for, 23–24, 24*f*
   syringes for, 19, 22, 22*f*

# H

# I

# M

Mealtime insulin. *See* Prandial (mealtime) insulin
Medication log, 53
Metformin, 38*f*
Multiple daily injections (MDI), 30–31, 30*t*, 39

# N

Needles, short *vs.* long, 25
Neutral protamine Hagedorn insulin. *See* NPH insulin
Niacinamide, insulin aspart with (Fiasp), 8*t*, 10, 20*t*
Novolin N, 8*t*, 20*t*. *See also* NPH insulin
Novolin R, 8*t*, 20*t*. *See also* Regular human insulin (U-100)
Novolin 70/30, 17*t*
Novolog, 20*t*
NovoLog, 8*t*, 10. *See also* Insulin aspart
NovoLog Mix 70/30, 17*t*
NPH insulin, 11–12
   agitation or mixing of, 11–12
   brand names, 8*t*, 20*t*
   cloudy appearance of, 11, 28
   comparative action of, 9*f*
   cost of, 12
   duration of action, 8*t*, 11–12
   mixing of (premixed products), 15–16, 17*t*
   onset of action, 8*t*
   purchase without prescription, 12
   regimen for type 1 diabetes, 30*t*
   in sample regimens
      four injections per day, 41–43, 42*f*, 43*f*
      three injections per day, 40, 41*f*
      two injections per day, 39, 40*f*
   storage of, 20*t*, 28
   time to peak action, 8*t*, 12

# O

# P